ANCIENT ENCYCLOPEDIA OF HERBAL MEDICINES

Unlock the Secrets of Ancient Remedies: A Comprehensive Guide to Herbal Plants, Natural Healing, and Traditional Medicine for Holistic Health and Wellness

RYAN T. GROVES

COPYRIGHT © 2024 BY RYAN T. GROVES

All rights reserved. No part of this publication may be reproduced, distributed, or transmitted in any form or by any means, including photocopying, recording, or other electronic or mechanical methods, without the prior written permission of the publisher, except in the case of brief quotations embodied in critical reviews and certain other noncommercial uses permitted by copyright law.

INTRODUCTION 6
   Herbal Medicine's History 6
   The Current Significance of Herbal Medicine ... 8
   Recognizing the Use of Herbal Medicine 9
   The Moral Aspects of Herbal Medicine 11
   Herbal Medicine's Future Directions 13
CHAPTER ONE 17
  BASICS OF BOTANY 17
   Anatomy and Physiology of Plants 17
   Categorization of Therapeutic Herbs 19
   Methods of Cultivation and Harvesting 21
   Sustainable Methods for Growing Herbs 23
   Preservation of Therapeutic Plant Types 26
CHAPTER TWO 30
EXAMINING THE SCIENCE OF MEDICINAL PLANTS WITH PHARMACOGNOSY 30
   Chemical Components of Therapeutic Plants. 31
   Standardization and Quality Assurance 35
   Pharmacological Examination of Herbal Supplements 37
   Herbal Product Side Effects and Toxicology ... 39

CHAPTER THREE 43

EXAMINING CONVENTIONAL HERBAL TREATMENTS 43

Native American Traditional Medicine 44

Customs in Traditional Medicine 46

Herbs in Various Cultures 47

Herbal Healing Ceremonies and Rituals 50

Transfer of Herbal Knowledge 52

CHAPTER FOUR 55

BRIDGING HERBAL MEDICINE AND MODERN SCIENCE: A COMPREHENSIVE EXPLORATION 55

Evidence-Based Herbal Therapy 58

Clinical Trials as well as Research Techniques 60

Herbal Compounds' Pharmacokinetics and Pharmacodynamics 62

The Molecular Underpinnings of Herbal Remedies 65

CHAPTER FIVE 69

INVESTIGATING HERBAL CONCOCTIONS AND USES 69

External Uses: Oils, Salves, and Poultices 71

Supplements with Herbs and Nutraceuticals .73

Herbal Personal Care and Cosmetic Items......75

Medicinal Herbs' Applications in Cooking and Gastronomy 76

CHAPTER SIX...79

INVESTIGATING HERBAL MEDICINE IN PARTICULAR HEALTH CONDITIONS...79

Herbal Remedies for Respiratory Conditions .80

Herbal Treatment of Intestinal Illnesses.........82

Herbal Therapy to Promote Heart Health 83

Using Herbs to Boost the Immune System 85

Herbal Remedies for Nervous System Disorders 87

CHAPTER SEVEN 90

GETTING AROUND THE LAW AND REGULATION FOR HERBAL PRODUCTS 90

Global Herbal Product Regulation 90

QA and GMPs (good manufacturing practices) 93

Traditional Knowledge and Intellectual Property Rights 95

Marketing Herbal Products with Integrity 97

Herbal medicine and consumer safety 99

INTRODUCTION

Herbal medicine, sometimes referred to as botanical medicine or phytotherapy, is the practice of treating a variety of illnesses and promoting health via the use of plants, plant extracts, and plant-based products. It is among the most ancient kind of medicine still used by human communities worldwide. Plants have always been an important source of therapeutic treatments, and their use is still very important in modern medicine. This thorough investigation will cover the background, significance, applications, moral dilemmas, and potential directions of herbal therapy.

Herbal Medicine's History

Herbal medicine has a long history, having been used by ancient Mesopotamians, Egyptians, Greeks, Romans, Chinese, and Indian civilizations, among others, for thousands of years. To cure ailments and preserve health, these cultures depended on indigenous plants and botanical knowledge that was passed down through the years.

Medical papyri from ancient Egypt, such as the Edwin Smith and Ebers papyri, record a wide range of herbal cures for different illnesses, indicating a highly developed knowledge of plant medicine. In a similar vein, the Greeks and Romans achieved important advances in herbal therapy. Authors such as Hippocrates and Dioscorides recorded the therapeutic benefits of plants in their works.

Herbal medicines are also widely used in Traditional Chinese Medicine (TCM) and Ayurveda, the traditional Indian medical system. While Ayurveda concentrates on the doshas—Vata, Pitta, and Kapha—and employs medicines to balance and harmonize the body, TCM emphasizes the harmony of Yin and Yang energies.

Herbal treatment was very popular in Europe throughout the Middle Ages, when monasteries were used as educational and growing centers for herbs. During this period, herbalists like Nicholas Culpeper and Hildegard of Bingen made important contributions to the field of herbalism.

With the advent of pharmaceutical medications and modern treatment, herbal medicine has seen a drop in popularity in recent times. But in recent decades, there has been a rebirth of interest in herbal therapy, driven by a greater realization of the drawbacks and adverse consequences of traditional treatments.

The Current Significance of Herbal Medicine

For a number of reasons, herbal medicine is still very important in modern medicine. First of all, a lot of individuals favor natural therapies over pharmaceutical ones since they are worried about the long-term health impacts and adverse effects of the latter. An alternative that is kinder and has fewer side effects is herbal medicine.

Second, people with little incomes or those living in isolated places with little access to contemporary medical facilities can obtain healthcare through herbal medicine. Compared to conventional drugs, traditional herbal medicines are frequently more accessible and less expensive.

Herbal medicine also provides a comprehensive approach to health, treating the body's underlying imbalances as well as symptoms. Numerous herbs have nutritional value in addition to their therapeutic qualities, which promote general health and wellbeing.

Furthermore, there is mounting scientific proof that some herbal medicines are effective for treating a range of illnesses. Numerous medicinal plants have been shown to have anti-inflammatory, antioxidant, antibacterial, and immunomodulatory qualities in studies.

Recognizing the Use of Herbal Medicine

There are many different customs and practices related to herbal medicine, and each one has its unique preparation and administration techniques. Typical herbal medication forms consist of:

1.Herbal Infusions and Teas: By steeping the plant material in hot water, many medicinal plants can be ingested as infusions or teas. By using this technique, medicinal ingredients can be extracted from the herbs without sacrificing their flavor.

2.Extracts and Tinctures: Plant material is soaked in glycerin or alcohol to create concentrated herbal extracts known as tinctures. Their extended shelf life and ease of use make them a popular choice.

3. Herbal poultices and compresses: To treat inflammation, discomfort, and other skin disorders, mashed or ground herbs are applied directly to the skin. Similar procedures are used in compresses, but instead of applying the decoction or infusion directly to the afflicted area, a cloth is soaked in it.

4. Tablets and Capsules: For convenient use, a variety of herbal supplements are offered in tablet or capsule form. Standardized extracts of particular plants are frequently included in these formulations to ensure uniform dosage.

5. Topical Preparations: For a variety of uses, such as pain management, skincare, and wound healing, herbal ointments, creams, and salves are applied directly to the skin.

6. Aromatherapy: Due to its therapeutic benefits for mood, stress, and physical problems, essential oils produced from fragrant plants are utilized in aromatherapy.

7. Customs: Native American tribes worldwide possess distinct customs around herbal medicine,

which are frequently transmitted verbally among successive generations. In addition to the use of medicinal herbs, these practices may also incorporate ceremonies, rituals, and spiritual elements.

Understanding pharmacology, botany, and conventional medical systems is necessary to comprehend the use of herbal medicine. Herbalists go through a rigorous training program to learn about the characteristics of various plants, how they interact with the body, and how to create potent cures.

The Moral Aspects of Herbal Medicine

Although there are many advantages to using herbal treatment, there are also moral issues to be aware of:

1.Sustainability: Since many medicinal plants are taken from their natural habitat, overharvesting and the depletion of natural resources are worries. The long-term availability of herbal treatments depends on conservation initiatives, medicinal plant production, and sustainable harvesting methods.

2.Safety and Quality: There can be a lot of variation in the quality of herbal goods, and problems like contamination, adulteration, and mislabeling can put customers at danger. In order to guarantee the safety and effectiveness of herbal products, quality control procedures, standardized testing, and regulation are required.

3.Cultural Appropriation: There are concerns regarding cultural appropriation when traditional herbal knowledge is commercialized without giving indigenous populations due credit or appreciation. Ethical herbal medicine methods must uphold the cultural legacy and intellectual property rights of indigenous peoples and traditional healers.

4.Informed Consent: In order to help patients make educated decisions, herbalists must accurately tell them of the possible advantages, hazards, and restrictions associated with using herbal treatments. Patients have a right to know why certain treatments are advised as well as how they might mix with prescription drugs.

5.Professional Integrity: Herbalists should follow professional guidelines for their work, which include continuing education, moral behavior, and openness when interacting with patients and other medical professionals. Maintaining honesty and responsibility helps people believe that herbal therapy is a valid kind of treatment.

To encourage responsible stewardship of medicinal plants and fair access to herbal healthcare, herbalists, researchers, regulators, and indigenous populations must work together to address these ethical considerations.

Herbal Medicine's Future Directions

Innovations in technology, changing healthcare requirements, and continuous research will influence the direction of herbal medicine in the future. In the upcoming years, the following trends are probably going to have an impact on how herbal medicine develops and is incorporated:

1.Scientific study: To investigate the effectiveness, safety, and mechanisms of action of herbal treatments, there is a growing interest in carrying out rigorous scientific study. Evidence-based practice is being made easier by developments in analytical methods, genomic research, and clinical trials, which are illuminating the therapeutic potential of medicinal plants.

2.Personalized Medicine: The significance of tailored treatment plans is becoming more widely acknowledged as precision medicine techniques gain traction. Herbal medicine presents the possibility of customized treatments based on heredity, metabolism, and lifestyle variables, enabling focused interventions catered to the individual requirements of the patient.

3.Integration with Conventional Medicine: Herbal medicine is becoming more and more accepted in conventional healthcare systems as scientific data demonstrating the effectiveness of certain of its therapies mounts. Integrative medicine methods, which provide patients a comprehensive approach to healthcare by fusing alternative therapies like herbal medicine with traditional treatments, are growing more popular.

4.Regulatory Frameworks: There are significant differences in the way herbal goods are regulated amongst nations, with some enforcing strict quality control standards and others having weak laws. Ensuring label transparency, putting quality assurance procedures into place, and harmonizing regulatory frameworks are critical to consumer safety and trust in herbal medicine.

5.Digital Health Technologies: Information on herbal medicine is being shared more and more through digital platforms and mobile applications, which may also be used to virtually consult with herbalists and make herbal goods easier to obtain. These technologies may enhance patient education, treatment adherence, and result monitoring for herbal remedies.

6.Cultivation and Sustainability: A trend is occurring toward the cultivation of medicinal herbs through sustainable agricultural methods, as worries about the sustainability of wild-harvested medicinal plants develop. To preserve natural environments, boost local economies, and conserve biodiversity, agroforestry, organic farming, and community-based projects are being encouraged.

To sum up, herbal medicine has a long history, plays a big role in modern healthcare, has a variety of applications, and its future is shaped by ethical issues. Herbal medicine will continue to develop as an important part of holistic healthcare, offering individualized, sustainable, and culturally sensitive methods of supporting health and healing, as scientific understanding and societal attitudes change.

CHAPTER ONE
BASICS OF BOTANY

The basic ideas and principles pertaining to plants, including their morphology, physiology, taxonomy, cultivation, and conservation, are covered by botanical basics. Anyone working in the field of herbal medicine, whether as a practitioner, researcher, or hobbyist, has to grasp these fundamentals. We will cover plant anatomy and physiology, classification of medicinal plants, cultivation and harvesting methods, sustainable herbal farming practices, and medicinal plant species conservation in this extensive investigation.

Anatomy and Physiology of Plants

Having specialized structures and functions tailored to their survival and reproduction, plants are multicellular, complex organisms. Some essential elements of plant anatomy and physiology are as follows:

1.Roots: The roots serve as the plant's anchor in the ground and take up water and nutrients from the surrounding soil. They might also hold onto reserves and carbs.

2.Stems: Between the roots and the leaves, stems carry nutrients, water, and photosynthates while also supporting the structure. They might also be used as places to store things and grow them vegetatively.

3.The main locations for photosynthesis, where chlorophyll-containing cells transform light energy into chemical energy, are leaves. They also control transpiration and gas exchange.

4.Flowers: Flowers are reproductive organs that use sexual reproduction to create seeds. They draw pollinators and make fertilization easier, which results in the development of fruits and seeds.

5.Fruits: Fertilized flowers give rise to fruits, which are seeds meant for distribution. They are essential for the wind or animals that disperse seeds, and they can have either fleshy or dry structures.

6.Seeds: Encased in protective seed coats, seeds are latent, embryonic plants. They have the genetic material required for germination and development into fully grown plants.

The study of plant functions and processes, such as photosynthesis, respiration, growth, development, and response to external stimuli, is known as plant physiology. A thorough understanding of plant physiology is necessary to maximize the quality and productivity of medicinal plants while refining cultivation techniques.

Categorization of Therapeutic Herbs

A wide range of species are utilized as medicinal plants because of their potential medical benefits. A number of factors, such as their pharmacological effects, traditional usage, phytochemical makeup, and botanical features, can be used to classify them. Medicinal plant classifications that are frequently used include:

1.Taxonomic Classification: Based on their botanical traits, such as family, genus, and species, medicinal plants can be grouped into many taxonomic categories. Herbs such as peppermint (Mentha ×

piperita) and rosemary (Rosmarinus officinalis) belong to the mint family (Lamiaceae).

2.Phytochemical Classification: Alkaloids, flavonoids, terpenoids, and phenolic compounds are only a few of the many bioactive substances found in medicinal plants. Their pharmacological characteristics and main phytochemical ingredients can be used to classify them. For instance, opium poppy (Papaver somniferum), a plant abundant in alkaloids, is utilized for its hypnotic and analgesic properties.

3.Traditional Classification: Medicinal plants are categorized according to their traditional usage and therapeutic indications in a number of traditional healing systems, including Traditional Chinese Medicine (TCM) and Ayurveda. For instance, TCM classifies herbs based on their energy qualities (hot, cold, warm, and cool) and how they affect particular meridians or organs.

4.Geographic Classification: The geographic distribution and natural habitats of medicinal plants can also be used to classify them. Indigenous societies have long utilized certain endemic plants, which are native to particular places. For instance, ginseng (Panax spp.), which is indigenous to East

Asia, is prized in traditional Asian medicine for its adaptogenic qualities.

Methods of Cultivation and Harvesting

The methods used for cultivation and harvesting medicinal plants are essential to guaranteeing their sustainability, quality, and productivity. When cultivating medicinal herbs, a number of aspects need to be taken into account, such as soil type, climate, availability of water, exposure to light, and insect control. Some popular growing and harvesting methods utilized in herbal medicine include the following:

1.Site Selection: Pick a location that is ideal, protected from severe weather and winds, has enough sunlight, and well-drained soil. Test the pH and nutritional levels of the soil, and make any necessary amendments to maximize plant growth.

2.Propagation: Depending on the species and propagation technique, propagate medicinal plants from seeds, cuttings, divisions, or tissue culture. For genetic purity and vigor, start with premium seeds or plant materials from reliable suppliers.

3.Planting: Considering the growth patterns and spacing requirements of medicinal herbs, plant them at the proper depth and spacing. Mulch around the plants helps control soil temperature, keep moisture in the soil, and discourage weed growth.

4.Watering: Apply enough water to the soil to maintain constant moisture levels, particularly in dry or hot weather. Steer clear of overwatering, which can cause root rot and other issues with water.

5.Fertilization: To enhance soil nutrients and encourage strong plant growth, apply organic or synthetic fertilizers as needed. To prevent nutrient imbalances and pollution of the environment, use fertilizers sparingly and according to prescribed application rates.

6.Control of Pests and Diseases: Keep an eye out for indications of pests, illnesses, and nutrient shortages in plants on a regular basis. To minimize pest damage and decrease reliance on synthetic chemicals, implement integrated pest management (IPM) options, such as crop rotation, companion planting, biological treatments, and organic pesticides.

7.Harvesting: To optimize the medicinal properties of plants and reduce post-harvest losses, harvest them at the right time of growth. Harvesting times vary based on the section of the plant (leaves, flowers, roots, etc.) that is used and the desired amount of bioactive components. To prevent harming the plants and contaminating the gathered material, use clean, sharp equipment.

Sustainable Methods for Growing Herbs

For medicinal plant species and ecosystems to be viable over the long term, sustainability in herbal agriculture is essential. Numerous medicinal plants are in danger of becoming extinct due to unsustainable harvesting methods, habitat damage, overexploitation, and climate change. Using sustainable farming methods is crucial for maintaining biodiversity, safeguarding natural ecosystems, and assisting regional communities. Some fundamental ideas of sustainable herbal farming are as follows:

1.Conservation of Biodiversity: Grow a wide variety of therapeutic plants to replicate natural ecosystems and improve resistance to pests, illnesses, and environmental stressors. In order to boost biodiversity and ecosystem services, steer clear of monoculture and instead encourage polyculture, intercropping, and agroforestry systems.

2.Native Plant Conservation: Give priority to cultivating native species of medicinal plants that are suited to the soil and climate of the area. By implementing programs for habitat conservation and restoration, protect and restore natural environments that are home to threatened or endangered plant species.

3.Adopting organic farming methods will help you reduce the amount of synthetic inputs you use, such as chemical pesticides, fertilizers, and herbicides. To increase soil fertility, structure, and biodiversity, use composting, crop rotation, cover crops, and organic soil additives.

4.Water Conservation: To maximize water use efficiency and minimize water consumption, put water-saving strategies into practice, such as drip irrigation, rainwater collection, and soil moisture monitoring. To prevent contamination and depletion of freshwater resources and aquatic ecosystems, practice water stewardship.

5.Energy Efficiency: By implementing energy-efficient technologies, such as solar-powered irrigation pumps, renewable energy systems, and energy-saving techniques, herbal farming can cut down on its energy usage and greenhouse gas emissions.

6.Managing Waste: Reduce the amount of waste produced and encourage the recycling, composting, and repurposing of organic materials, including crop leftovers, pruning debris, and packaging materials. Put waste management techniques into practice to lessen pollution to the environment and encourage resource conservation.

7.Involve stakeholders, local communities, and indigenous peoples in decision-making processes pertaining to the production and preservation of herbal remedies. Encourage partnerships, cooperatives, and community-based projects that empower underprivileged people and advance sustainable lives.

Preservation of Therapeutic Plant Types

In order to prevent the loss of medicinal plant species and maintain their genetic variety for future generations, conservation initiatives are crucial. The existence of medicinal plants is threatened by a number of reasons, such as pollution, invasive species, deforestation, overharvesting, habitat loss, and climate change. The goals of conservation strategies are to mitigate these risks and advance the long-term administration of resources related to medicinal plants. Some important strategies for the preservation of species of medicinal plants are as follows:

1.Protected Areas: To preserve natural habitats and endangered plant species, establish protected areas such as national parks, nature reserves, and botanical gardens. Put policies in place to stop poaching, illegal logging, habitat degradation, and other types of exploitation inside protected areas.

2.The goal of in situ conservation is to maintain medicinal plant species in their natural environments. Examples of such methods include land acquisition, protected area management, habitat restoration, and biodiversity conservation initiatives. To evaluate population dynamics, habitat quality, and threats to plant species, carry out ecological study and monitoring.

3.Ex Situ Conservation: To protect medicinal plant species away from their natural environments, establish ex situ conservation institutions, such as living collections, botanical gardens, seed banks, and germplasm repositories. Gather and store plant tissues, seeds, and genetic material for use in upcoming studies, propagations, and reintroduction projects.

4.Species Recovery Plans: Work with local communities, government agencies, and conservation organizations to develop conservation strategies and plans for endangered or threatened species of medicinal plants. Put policies in place to lessen risks, rebuild ecosystems, resolve disputes amicably, and keep an eye on population trends.

5.Community-Based Conservation: By using participatory methods, traditional knowledge exchange, and capacity-building programs, involve local communities, indigenous peoples, and traditional healers in conservation activities. Acknowledge and honor indigenous rights, customs, and ecological knowledge pertaining to medicinal plants.

6.Policy and Regulation: Pass and implement laws, rules, and policies that guard against overexploitation, illicit trading, and unsustainable harvesting methods for medicinal plant species and their environments. To encourage conservation and ethical sourcing, promote fair trade agreements, certification programs, and sustainable management techniques.

7.Education and Awareness: Spread knowledge among the general population about the value of protecting medicinal plants, sustainable harvesting methods, and the contribution of biodiversity to human health and welfare. Offer outreach initiatives, educational resources, and training to encourage communities and stakeholders to get involved in conservation activities.

To sum up, the knowledge of plant anatomy, physiology, classification, cultivation, and conservation that is pertinent to the practice of herbal medicine is included in the area of botanical basics. We can encourage the ethical use and preservation of medicinal plant resources for the benefit of current and future generations by comprehending these core ideas and implementing sustainable practices.

CHAPTER TWO

EXAMINING THE SCIENCE OF MEDICINAL PLANTS WITH PHARMACOGNOSY

The study of natural compounds derived from plants, fungi, and other organisms, with an emphasis on their pharmacological characteristics, chemical makeup, and therapeutic potential, is the multidisciplinary discipline of pharmacognosy. It is essential to the discovery, creation, and assurance of the quality of herbal remedies. We will delve into the complexities of pharmacognosy in this in-depth investigation, covering subjects like the chemical makeup of medicinal plants, methods of extraction and formulation, quality assurance and standardization, pharmacological screening of herbal extracts, and the toxicology and side effects of herbal products.

Chemical Components of Therapeutic Plants

A wide range of bioactive substances found in medicinal plants support their therapeutic benefits. These chemical components fall into a number of general types, including as polysaccharides, essential oils, phenolic compounds, terpenoids, flavonoids, and alkaloids. Every class of chemicals has distinct modes of action and pharmacological characteristics. As an illustration:

1.Alkaloids: These nitrogen-containing substances have a variety of pharmacological properties, including sedative, analgesic, antipyretic, and anti-inflammatory actions. Alkaloid-rich medicinal plants include cinchona (Cinchona spp.), a source of quinine used to treat malaria, and opium poppy (Papaver somniferum), which contains morphine and codeine.

2.Flavonoids: Fruits, vegetables, and medicinal plants contain flavonoids, which are polyphenolic chemicals. They have cardioprotective, anti-inflammatory, anticancer, and antioxidant qualities. Flavonoid-rich medicinal plants include St. John's wort (Hypericum perforatum), which is used to treat anxiety and depression, and ginkgo biloba, which is well-known for its neuroprotective properties.

3.Terpenoids: Made from isoprene units, terpenoids—also referred to as terpenes or essential oils—are fragrant chemicals. Their pharmacological properties are multifaceted, encompassing antibacterial, antiviral, antifungal, and anti-inflammatory properties. Mentha spp. are medicinal plants that are rich in terpenoid compounds. (mint), which is high in menthol, which has cooling and analgesic effects, and Artemisia annua, or sweet wormwood, which is high in artemisinin and is used to cure malaria.

4.Phenolic Compounds: Found in a wide variety of fruits, vegetables, and medicinal plants, phenolic compounds are antioxidants. They offer defense against inflammation, oxidative stress, and long-term illnesses. Green tea (Camellia sinensis), which is prized for its catechin concentration, and Echinacea spp., which are believed to boost the immune system and ward off colds, are two examples of medicinal plants high in phenolics.

5.Polysaccharides: Complex carbohydrates called polysaccharides are present in the mucilages, gums, and cell walls of plants. They possess antioxidant, anti-inflammatory, and immunomodulatory qualities. Medicinal plants high in polysaccharides include Aloe vera, which is well-known for its ability to heal wounds, and Astragalus membranaceus, which is utilized in traditional Chinese medicine for its immune-boosting qualities.

Methods of Formulation and Extraction

Specialized methods are needed to extract bioactive components from medicinal plants in a way that maximizes purity, potency, and production. Typical techniques for extraction consist of:

1.Maceration: To extract soluble chemicals, plant material is soaked in a solvent, such as water, alcohol, or oil. It is an easy-to-use and reasonably priced technique that can be used to extract a variety of phytochemicals.

2.Percolation: This dynamic extraction technique includes regulating the temperature, pressure, and flow rate of a solvent as it passes through a bed of powdered plant material. It minimizes solvent consumption and extraction time while enabling effective extraction of active components.

3.Soxhlet Extraction: This continuous extraction technique cycles a solvent between a condenser and a heated flask containing the plant material until equilibrium is achieved. It is frequently employed to remove lipophilic substances from plant sources.

4.Supercritical Fluid Extraction (SFE): SFE extracts non-polar and semi-polar chemicals from plant materials by using supercritical fluids as solvents, such as carbon dioxide (CO_2). It has benefits including easy solvent cleanup, minimal environmental effect, and selective extraction.

5.Steam Distillation: This method is used to extract volatile substances from aromatic plant components, such as essential oils. The process entails vaporizing and condensing the volatile components into a liquid by flowing steam through the plant material.

Depending on their intended application and mode of administration, bioactive substances can be extracted and then made into a variety of dosage forms, including tinctures, extracts, capsules, pills, ointments, lotions, and teas. Formulation approaches are designed to ensure patient safety and compliance while optimizing the stability, bioavailability, and efficacy of herbal medications.

Standardization and Quality Assurance

To guarantee the security, effectiveness, and uniformity of herbal products, quality control and standardization are crucial components of herbal therapy. In order to ensure that the final goods and manufacturing processes satisfy the required standards and requirements, quality control techniques entail evaluating raw materials. Important components of standardization and quality assurance consist of:

1. Botanical Identification: To avoid adulteration, mislabeling, and contamination of herbal products, it is essential to accurately identify plant species and plant parts. Techniques for botanical identification include chemical analysis, chromatographic fingerprinting, DNA barcoding, and macroscopic and microscopic inspection.

2. Physicochemical study: This type of study examines the moisture content, ash value, extractable matter, solvent residues, heavy metals, microbiological contamination, and pesticide residues of herbal materials and extracts. Mass spectrometry,

chromatography, spectrophotometry, titration, and gravimetric analysis are examples of analytical techniques.

3.Biochemical Analysis: Using quantitative tests and chemical profiling techniques, biochemical analysis determines the concentration of bioactive chemicals in herbal extracts, including phenolic compounds, alkaloids, flavonoids, and terpenoids. The results of these tests reveal details regarding the content and effectiveness of herbal items.

4.Pharmacological Screening: Using both in vitro and in vivo experiments, pharmacological screening assesses the pharmacological characteristics and biological activities of herbal extracts. To confirm conventional applications and pinpoint possible therapeutic targets, pharmacological studies evaluate characteristics including antioxidant activity, anti-inflammatory activity, antibacterial activity, analgesic activity, and cytotoxicity.

5.Standardization: According to scientific data, legal needs, and conventional wisdom, standards and criteria are developed for the identity, purity, potency, and quality of herbal products. Quantifying marker molecules, creating chemical profiles, and creating reference materials and standards for comparison are examples of standardization techniques.

Pharmacological Examination of Herbal Supplements

In the process of finding and developing new drugs, pharmacological screening is an essential phase that helps uncover possible therapeutic molecules from natural sources, such medicinal plants. A range of experimental models and tests are used to assess the pharmacological properties of herbal extracts. Typical pharmacological screening techniques include the following:

1.Antioxidant Activity: Herbal extracts' capacity to scavenge free radicals and prevent oxidative stress is measured by antioxidant assays. The ABTS (2,2'-azino-bis(3-ethylbenzothiazoline-6-sulfonic acid)) radical scavenging assay, the DPPH (2,2-diphenyl-1-picrylhydrazyl) radical scavenging assay, and the FRAP (ferric reducing antioxidant power) assay are common assays.

2.Anti-Inflammatory Activity: Assays for reducing inflammation assess a herbal extract's capacity to obstruct inflammatory mediators and pathways. Pro-inflammatory cytokines like TNF-α (tumor necrosis factor-alpha) and IL-6 (interleukin-6) as well as enzymes like COX-2 (cyclooxygenase-2) and LOX (lipoxygenase) are frequently inhibited in experiments.

3.Antimicrobial Activity: Herbal extracts' capacity to prevent the growth of harmful microbes like bacteria, fungus, and viruses is measured by antimicrobial assays. The broth dilution method, the disk diffusion method, and the agar diffusion method are common assays.

4.Anticancer Activity: Cytotoxicity and anticancer effects of herbal extracts against tumor models and cancer cell lines are assessed using anticancer assays. The xenograft model, the clonogenic assay, and the MTT (3-(4,5-dimethylthiazol-2-yl)-2,5-diphenyltetrazolium bromide) assay are examples of common assays.

5.Neuroprotective Activity: Tests for neuroprotection determine if herbal extracts can shield neurons from excitotoxicity, oxidative stress, and neurodegeneration. Neurotransmitter release, apoptosis, and neuronal viability are measured using common techniques.

Pharmacological screening aids in the prioritization of candidates for additional preclinical and clinical research and offers insightful information about the possible therapeutic applications of herbal extracts. It also advances knowledge of the mechanisms of action that underlie the pharmacological effects of therapeutic plants.

Herbal Product Side Effects and Toxicology

Even while herbal remedies are usually regarded as safe when used as directed, there are situations in which they can be poisonous or have unfavorable consequences. Medication interactions, allergic reactions, incorrect dosage, contamination, or adulteration of herbal items can all lead to adverse effects. Overdosing, mishandling, or the presence of hazardous substances in herbal remedies can all result in toxicity. The following are typical side effects and toxicological issues connected to herbal products:

1.Drug-Herb Interactions: Herbal products may influence the metabolism, effectiveness, and toxicity of prescription pharmaceuticals, over-the-counter treatments, and nutritional supplements. medication-herb interactions can interfere with medication absorption, distribution, metabolism, or excretion. They can also intensify or suppress the effects of drugs, induce the activity of enzymes involved in drug metabolism, and more.

2.Allergic Reactions: Skin rashes, itching, hives, swelling, respiratory symptoms, gastrointestinal problems, or anaphylaxis are some of the signs that can indicate an allergic reaction to herbal products. Plants in the Asteraceae family (ragweed, chamomile), Apiaceae family (celery, parsley), and Lamiaceae family (mint, basil) are common allergic plants.

3.hazardous Compounds: A number of therapeutic plants contain compounds that, when taken in large quantities or over an extended period of time, can have hazardous consequences. These compounds include pyrrolizidine alkaloids, glycosides, saponins, cyanogenic glycosides, and alkaloids. Plants that are poisonous include Aconitum spp. (aconite), species of Digitalis. (foxglove) and the deadly nightshade, Atropa belladonna.

4.Contamination and Adulteration: During cultivation, harvesting, processing, storage, or distribution, herbal products may get polluted with heavy metals, fungicides, herbicides, microbial pathogens, or other contaminants. Another frequent issue is the adulteration of herbal goods with unreported or subpar substances, especially in the international herbal trade.

5.Misuse and Overdose: When herbal products are misused or overdosed, it can have harmful consequences or even be toxic, especially in sensitive groups including children, the elderly, pregnant women, and people with underlying medical issues. Herbal items such as stimulant herbs (like Ephedra spp., Ma Huang) and psychoactive herbs (like Kratom, Salvia divinorum) have the potential to be abused or overdosed.

Utilizing in vitro and in vivo models, toxicological studies analyze the safety profile of herbal products by determining their genotoxicity, carcinogenicity, acute, subacute, and chronic toxicity as well as their developmental and reproductive toxicity. These studies offer important information for evaluating safety, assessing risks, and making regulatory decisions about the use of herbal medicines.

To sum up, pharmacognosy is the study of medicinal plants from the viewpoints of chemistry, pharmacology, and toxicology. To guarantee the efficacy, safety, and quality of herbal products, one must be aware of their chemical composition, extraction methods, quality control procedures, pharmacological characteristics, and safety issues. Researchers, medical professionals, and regulators can encourage the ethical use and evidence-based integration of herbal medicines into global healthcare systems by incorporating pharmacognostic principles into herbal medicine practice.

CHAPTER THREE
EXAMINING CONVENTIONAL HERBAL TREATMENTS

Herbal treatments with a deep history comprise a diverse range of healing techniques that have been handed down through the ages in many different societies and civilizations across the globe. These treatments, which have their roots in folklore, indigenous wisdom, and cultural legacy, demonstrate a close relationship to the natural world and the ancestors' understanding of herbal medicine. We will delve into the complexities of traditional herbal medicines in this thorough examination, covering indigenous healing techniques, folk medicine traditions, herbalism in various cultures, herbal healing rituals and ceremonies, and the dissemination of herbal knowledge.

Native American Traditional Medicine

Native Americans' spiritual beliefs, cultural rituals, and ecological expertise are intricately entwined with their healing practices. They include an all-encompassing strategy for health and wellness that takes into account the connections between people, the natural world, and the universe. Native American healers, sometimes referred to as shamans, medicine men, or medicine women, are essential in leading healing rites and ceremonies that make use of sacred artifacts, medicinal herbs, and ceremonial techniques.

1.Sacred Plants: Certain plants have long been valued by indigenous cultures as sacred partners with strong therapeutic qualities. In ceremonial settings, these sacred plants are employed to promote spiritual transformation, healing, and connection. Examples include the use of peyote (Lophophora williamsii) in Native American traditions, iboga (Tabernanthe iboga) in African spiritual practices, and ayahuasca (Banisteriopsis caapi) in Amazonian shamanism.

2.Spiritual Healing: Indigenous healing techniques frequently entail spiritual rites and ceremonies meant to bring balance and harmony back to the individual, the community, and the environment. Invoking healing energies, ancestral spirits, and divine forces, healing ceremonies may involve drumming, chanting, dancing, smudging, and storytelling.

3.Plant Medicine: In indigenous societies, plants are revered as spiritual teachers and allies that offer not only physical healing but also spiritual direction and insight. Native American healers employ a wide variety of medicinal plants, each with special qualities and therapeutic benefits. Plant medicines can be made and used as teas, tinctures, poultices, ceremonial brews, and other forms.

4.Cultural Continuity: Oral traditions, intergenerational knowledge transfer, and cultural continuity are fundamental to indigenous healing techniques. The elders are essential in maintaining and transmitting to the next generation the customs of healing, which helps indigenous cultures endure and adapt to social, economic, and environmental difficulties.

Customs in Traditional Medicine

Localized healing systems known as folk medicine traditions have developed within certain cultural contexts; these contexts are frequently rural or distant areas with limited access to modern healthcare. In order to cure common ailments and promote health and well-being, folk remedies draw on the collective wisdom of local healers, herbalists, midwives, and traditional practitioners who rely on indigenous plants, medicines, and rituals.

1.Home Remedies: Self-care and home remedies utilizing easily accessible plants, foods, and household items are frequently highlighted in folk medical traditions. Herbal teas, compresses, poultices, and topical preparations are examples of home remedies that can be used to treat skin illnesses, digestive issues, respiratory problems, and minor injuries.

2.Seasonal Practices: The practices of folk medicine are adapted to the cycles of the natural world and the varying seasons, with particular cures and customs designed for each season. Herbal harvests, planting ceremonies, cleansing rites, and seasonal detoxification programs are a few examples of seasonal practices that help the body and spirit harmonize with the cycles of nature.

3.Community Healing: Folk medicine has its roots in social solidarity and community networks. Healing procedures are frequently carried out in the framework of familial, kinship, and communal support. Local herbalists, wise women, and community healers are essential in helping their neighbors and fellow community members by offering medical care, spiritual direction, and emotional support.

4.Cultural Heritage: Each community's distinct history, set of values, and worldview are reflected in its folk medicine traditions, which are an essential component of its cultural heritage and identity. Oral traditions, folklore, and cultural practices are the means by which folk remedies are transmitted, safeguarding indigenous wisdom and ancestors' knowledge for posterity.

Herbs in Various Cultures

The use of plants for therapeutic purposes, or herbalism, is a widespread practice that has been observed in many cultures and civilizations worldwide. The fundamental ideas of herbalism—harnessing nature's therapeutic power to promote health, energy, and balance—remain constant, despite cultural variations in the particular plants, cures, and healing rituals used. Let's examine herbalism in many societies:

1.Traditional Chinese Medicine (TCM): With a history spanning thousands of years, TCM is among the most extensive and ancient systems of herbal medicine. The theory of Qi, or vital energy, and the equilibrium of Yin and Yang energies within the body are central to TCM. In TCM, herbal formulas are recommended based on the concepts of herbal energetics, individual constitution, and pattern diagnosis.

2.Ayurveda: With over 5,000 years of history, Ayurveda is the traditional medicinal system of India. According to Ayurvedic medicine, being healthy is about having a balanced body, mind, and soul. In Ayurveda, herbal treatments are categorized based on each person's dosha (constitutional type), taste (rasa), energy (virya), and post-digestive effect (vipaka).

3.Native American Herbal Medicine: Native Americans in North and South America utilize a wide range of traditional herbal medicines. Herbal remedies are used for medicinal purposes, ceremonial purposes, and spiritual purification. They are made from native plants such sweetgrass, cedar, tobacco, and sage.

4.European Herbalism: With roots in classical Greece and Rome, European herbalism boasts a long and distinguished history. European herbal traditions cover a broad spectrum of applications, from contemporary phytotherapy and plant medicine to folk medicine and alchemy from the Middle Ages. Plants with medicinal qualities, like chamomile, elderberry, yarrow, and valerian, have long been used by European herbalists.

5.African Herbalism: Native American communities all around the African continent utilize a variety of herbal remedies. A wide variety of plants, including neem, moringa, baobab, and hoodia, are used in herbal medicines. African herbalists employ plants to cure a variety of illnesses, such as skin diseases, reproductive health difficulties, malaria, and digestive disorders.

Herbal Healing Ceremonies and Rituals

In traditional herbal medicine, rituals and ceremonies are important components that facilitate spiritual connection, cultural expression, and healing transformation. Herbal medicine gains efficacy and potency via rituals that imbue it with spiritual significance and intention. Let's examine a few typical herbal healing rites and ceremonies:

1.Plant Spirit Medicine: A lot of traditional therapeutic practices acknowledge the "spirit" or spiritual nature of plants and aim to create a strong bond with the plant kingdom via prayers, offerings, and rituals. Plant spirit medicine is connecting with plant awareness, asking the spirits of the plants for direction, and accepting their healing benefits.

2.Plant Blessing Ceremonies: These are customs carried out to respect and call upon the blessings of therapeutic plants for recovery, defense, and enlightenment. Offerings of holy herbs, songs, prayers, and invocations to ancestors, nature deities, and plant spirits may all be a part of these ceremonies.

3.Herbal Harvest Ritual: Gathering medicinal plants, herbs, and botanicals from cultivated gardens or the wild is the occasion for ceremonial herbal harvests. These customs ask permission from the land spirits, thank the plants for their medicinal offerings, and guarantee sustainable harvesting methods that preserve biodiversity and ecological balance.

4.Medicine Making Ceremony: A spiritual and purposeful process of preparing herbal cures, tinctures, teas, and potions is included in medicine making rituals. To give the medicines healing energy and spiritual efficacy, these ceremonies may include rituals like drumming, chanting, smudging, and visualization.

5.Healing Circles: In a loving and encouraging setting, people join in healing circles to share their goals, prayers, and desires for transformation. Sacred spaces for healing, transformation, and group empowerment are created via the sharing and passing of herbal remedies, plant allies, and healing practices around the circle.

Transfer of Herbal Knowledge

One important and time-honored tradition that guarantees the continuation and preservation of conventional medical methods is the passing down of herbal knowledge from generation to generation. Oral traditions, apprenticeship relationships, experiential learning, and firsthand plant encounter are the usual methods used to impart herbal knowledge. Let's examine some typical approaches to the dissemination of herbal knowledge:

1.Oral Traditions: Elders, healers, and traditional practitioners in many indigenous societies transmit herbal knowledge verbally to younger generations. Stories, myths, tales, and songs that explain the therapeutic qualities, applications, and spiritual importance of medicinal herbs are all part of oral traditions.

2.Apprenticeship: In this age-old approach to studying herbalism, prospective herbalists are trained practically under the guidance of seasoned practitioners. Apprentices collaborate closely with their mentors, taking part in all facets of herbal practice, from harvesting and identifying plants to preparing medicines and performing healing ceremonies.

3.Experiential Learning: Building personal relationships, experimenting, and observing plants firsthand are all common ways that people learn about herbs. Aspiring herbalists spend time in the outdoors, developing a close relationship with the plant kingdom and refining their sense of smell and intuition.

4.Community Learning: Through get-togethers, workshops, lectures, and herbal conferences, communities exchange and share knowledge about herbs. Herbalists, healers, and plant enthusiasts can get together, network, and share their knowledge, experiences, and ideas at community learning events.

5.Written Texts: Manuscripts, written texts, and herbal compendiums act as archives for herbal knowledge, safeguarding for the benefit of future generations ancient cures, plant legends, and medicinal techniques. In their respective medical traditions, ancient writings like the "Yellow

Emperor's Classic of Internal Medicine" in Chinese medicine and the "Charaka Samhita" and "Sushruta Samhita" in Ayurveda are highly regarded as foundational texts.

Traditional herbal medicine will be preserved and thrive for future generations if we respect and preserve these age-old systems of information transfer. We strengthen our grasp of the therapeutic potential of plants and foster a closer bond with the natural world via the ongoing sharing of knowledge, expertise, and respect for the natural world.

CHAPTER FOUR

BRIDGING HERBAL MEDICINE AND MODERN SCIENCE: A COMPREHENSIVE EXPLORATION

Herbal medicine's incorporation into modern healthcare signifies the meeting point of traditional knowledge and cutting-edge research. Growing proof of the therapeutic value of medicinal plants and herbal treatments has been the driving force for further research, clinical trials, and evidence-based practice in the field of herbal medicine in recent years. The integration of herbal medicine into contemporary healthcare, evidence-based herbal medicine, clinical trials and research methodologies, pharmacokinetics and pharmacodynamics of herbal substances, and the molecular mechanisms of herbal activities will all be covered in detail in this examination.

Herbal medicine's incorporation into contemporary healthcare

Incorporating traditional herbal medicines and practices into contemporary medical settings, like hospitals, clinics, and primary care settings, is the process of integrating herbal medicine into modern healthcare. The usefulness of herbal medicine as a complementary and alternative therapy that can improve patient care, support holistic health, and increase treatment alternatives is acknowledged by this integrative approach. An essential component of incorporating herbal therapy into contemporary treatment is:

1.Multidisciplinary Collaboration: Physicians, pharmacists, herbalists, naturopathic doctors, and other allied health professionals must work together to integrate herbal therapy into contemporary healthcare. In order to create complete treatment programs that combine traditional therapies with herbal remedies specific to each patient's needs, multidisciplinary teams collaborate.

2.Patient-Centered Care: Integrative healthcare places a strong emphasis on a patient-centered strategy that gives the patient's preferences, values, and beliefs top priority when choosing a course of treatment. Healthcare professionals enable patients to make educated decisions about their healthcare alternatives, involve them in shared decision-making, and advise them of the dangers and advantages of herbal medicine.

3.Evidence-Based Practice: The foundation of integrative healthcare is evidence-based practice, which combines patient preferences, clinician judgment, and the best available scientific data. Healthcare professionals assess the quality, safety, and efficacy of herbal therapies and use the results to guide clinical decision-making through rigorous research, clinical trials, systematic reviews, and meta-analyses.

4.Safety and Quality Control: Integrative medicine places a high priority on patient safety and quality control by making sure that herbal products adhere to predetermined guidelines for safety, potency, and purity. In order to reduce the risk of adverse reactions and drug interactions, healthcare providers inform patients about the significance of choosing reliable sources, standardized goods, and evidence-based dosing guidelines.

5.Education and Training: To deliver integrative healthcare, medical professionals must get instruction and training in herbal medicine, botanical pharmacology, and integrative therapies. Opportunities to improve knowledge and abilities in the practice of herbal medicine are offered to healthcare professionals through workshops, certification courses, and continuing education programs.

Evidence-Based Herbal Therapy

Evidence-based herbal medicine is a medical strategy that prioritizes the application of scientific evidence to inform the choice, administration, and assessment of herbal treatments. The integration of modern research approaches with traditional knowledge enables the assessment of the safety, effectiveness, and clinical utility of herbal remedies for certain medical diseases. Essential tenets of evidence-based herbal medicine consist of:

1.Systematic Review: A systematic review is an extensive analysis of the literature that summarizes the conclusions of several research on a given subject or intervention. A transparent and rigorous approach to assessing the quality and strength of evidence supporting herbal therapies and pinpointing gaps in the body of research is to conduct systematic reviews.

2. The gold standard for assessing the safety and effectiveness of healthcare interventions, including herbal therapies, is a randomized controlled trial (RCT). Randomized controlled trials (RCTs) entail the random assignment of participants to treatment and control groups, the delivery of the intervention, and a comparison of group outcomes to evaluate effectiveness.

3. Meta-analysis is a statistical method that yields summary estimates of treatment effects by combining and analyzing data from several trials. When compared to individual trials, meta-analyses offer a quantitative synthesis of the data, enabling researchers to make more reliable judgments regarding the efficacy and safety of herbal therapies.

4. Observational Studies: Cohort and case-control studies are examples of observational studies that look at the relationship between exposure to herbs and health outcomes in actual environments. Even while observational studies are unable to prove

causation, they can offer important information about the long-term impacts, safety profile, and efficacy of herbal medicines in actual situations.

5.Pharmacological Research: Using both in vitro and in vivo experimental models, pharmacological research aims to understand the pharmacokinetics, pharmacodynamics, and mechanisms of action of herbal substances. Mechanistic insights into the therapeutic characteristics of herbal medicines are provided by pharmacological research, which clarify the biochemical processes, receptor interactions, and physiological impacts of these therapies.

Clinical Trials as well as Research Techniques

To assess the efficacy, safety, and practicality of herbal treatments in clinical settings, clinical studies are necessary. They offer a methodical and exacting structure for producing evidence, putting theories to the test, and guiding clinical judgment. Important factors to take into account when planning and carrying out herbal medicine clinical trials are:

1.Study Design: A variety of study designs, such as parallel-group RCTs, crossover trials, factorial trials, and pragmatic trials, may be used in clinical trials of herbal medicine. The research question, study objectives, demographic characteristics, and ethical considerations are some of the elements that influence the choice of study design.

2.Participant Selection: To guarantee the inclusion of eligible participants and the exclusion of those with contraindications or comorbidities that could skew the results, participant selection criteria for clinical studies using herbal medicine should be precisely specified. Targeted outreach, community involvement, and partnership with healthcare practitioners are a few examples of recruitment tactics.

3.Intervention: Standardized, well-characterized, and provided in accordance with evidence-based dose regimens are the best practices for herbal interventions in clinical studies. Testing for quality control is necessary to ensure that herbal products are consistent, pure, potent, and identifiable. The effectiveness of herbal medicines in comparison to established therapies or placebo is frequently assessed through the use of placebo-controlled trials and active comparator trials.

4.Clinical endpoints, such as symptom severity, disease progression, quality of life, and patient-reported outcomes, as well as objective measurements, such as biomarkers, laboratory testing, and imaging investigations, may be used as outcome measures in herbal medicine clinical trials. Tools for assessing outcomes should be sensitive to changes in health status, valid, and dependable.

5.Data analysis: Statistical techniques are used in clinical trials of herbal medicine to compare treatment groups, estimate treatment effectiveness, and evaluate safety results. Treatment adherence, heterogeneity of treatment effects, and missing data can all be taken into account via statistical approaches including intention-to-treat analysis, per-protocol analysis, and subgroup analysis.

Herbal Compounds' Pharmacokinetics and Pharmacodynamics

Basic ideas in pharmacology, pharmacokinetics and pharmacodynamics explain how medications are absorbed, distributed, metabolized, and excreted (ADME) as well as how they affect the body. To maximize the therapeutic benefits of herbal components and reduce the likelihood of negative side effects, it is crucial to comprehend their pharmacokinetic and pharmacodynamic features. The following factors are crucial to the pharmacokinetics and pharmacodynamics of herbal compounds:

1.The process by which herbal chemicals enter the bloodstream and make their way to the intended tissues after being administered is referred to as absorption. Herbal components can be taken by a number of different methods, such as injection, topical application, inhalation, and oral consumption. The chemical makeup of the molecule, the features of the formulation, and physiological aspects like intestinal permeability and gastric emptying all have an impact on absorption.

2.Distribution: The term "distribution" describes how the circulation carries herbal compounds throughout the body and how they build up in different tissues and organs. Blood flow, tissue perfusion, plasma protein binding, and the compound's physicochemical characteristics are some of the variables that affect distribution. Herbal chemicals have the potential to disperse widely to their intended locations of action or to collect in particular organs including the brain, kidneys, and liver.

3.The process by which enzymes in the liver and other tissues biotransform herbal substances to create metabolites that are more readily absorbed by the body and less soluble in water is known as metabolism. Herbal compounds may become active or inactive as a result of metabolism, or they may become inert. The metabolism of herbal compounds is significantly influenced by phase II conjugation enzymes, cytochrome P450 enzymes, and gut flora.

4.Excretion: The removal of herbal components and their metabolites from the body through perspiration, breath, urine, and other excretory pathways is referred to as excretion. Renal, biliary, and pulmonary excretion are examples of excretion pathways. Urinary pH, hepatic and renal function, and drug interactions are some of the factors that affect excretion rate and extent.

5.Pharmacodynamics: This term describes the physiological and biochemical impacts of herbal compounds on the body, as well as their side effects and mode of action. Various methods, including receptor binding, enzyme inhibition, ion channel modulation, and signal transduction pathways, may be employed by herbal substances to achieve their pharmacological effects. Pharmacodynamic investigations clarify the beginning of action, duration of effect, and dose-response correlations of herbal treatments.

The Molecular Underpinnings of Herbal Remedies

The biochemical interactions between herbal substances and cellular targets inside the body are the molecular mechanisms by which herbal medicines function to provide therapeutic effects on physiological processes, biochemical pathways, and disease states. Comprehending the molecular mechanisms underlying the effects of herbal remedies is essential to clarifying the medical value of plants and creating new treatments. Among the main molecular pathways by which herbs work are:

1.Receptor Binding: A number of herbal substances modulate signaling pathways and physiological responses by binding to particular receptors on cell surfaces or within cells. This process is how they achieve their pharmacological effects. Alkaloids binding to neurotransmitter receptors, phytoestrogens binding to estrogen receptors, and cannabinoids binding to cannabinoid receptors are a few examples.

2.Enzyme Inhibition: Herbal remedies have the ability to inhibit enzymes that are involved in signal transduction, metabolic pathways, and cellular activities. This can modify physiological responses as well as biochemical reactions. Examples include alkaloids that inhibit acetylcholinesterase and polyphenols that inhibit cyclooxygenase enzymes (COX). Protease inhibitors also inactivate viral proteases.

3.Ion Channel Modulation: The activity of ion channels in cell membranes can be modulated by herbal substances, which in turn controls how ions like calcium, chloride, sodium, and potassium move across the membrane. Ion channel modulation can affect the release of neurotransmitters, heart function, muscular contraction, and neuronal excitability. Terpenoids that modulate voltage-gated ion channels and flavonoids that modulate calcium channels are two examples.

4.Herbal remedies have the ability to stimulate or inhibit intracellular signaling pathways that are important in gene expression, protein synthesis, and cellular communication. Numerous physiological processes, such as immune response, apoptosis, differentiation, and cell proliferation, are mediated via signal transduction pathways. Examples include polyphenols blocking NF-κB (nuclear factor kappa-light-chain-enhancer of activated B cells) signaling and flavonoids stimulating the MAPK (mitogen-activated protein kinase) pathway.

5.Epigenetic Regulation: By modifying DNA methylation, histone changes, and non-coding RNA expression, herbal remedies may have an epigenetic impact on gene expression. Disease progression, cellular differentiation, and development can all be impacted by epigenetic control. Heterpenoids influencing microRNA expression, flavonoids controlling DNA methylation, and polyphenols controlling histone acetylation are a few examples.

Researchers can identify new therapeutic targets, improve herbal formulations, and create evidence-based interventions for a variety of medical problems by clarifying the molecular mechanisms underlying the activities of herbs. Molecular pharmacology techniques, including high-throughput screening, computer modeling, and molecular docking, make it easier to find and create herbal medications with improved safety, efficacy, and specificity.

To sum up, the incorporation of herbal medicine into contemporary healthcare signifies a vibrant collaboration between conventional knowledge and cutting-edge research. Evidence-based herbal medicine advances our knowledge of the therapeutic potential of medicinal plants and enhances patient care by fusing the scientific methods of current research with the holistic principles of herbalism. We can harness the healing power of nature to enhance resilience, health, and well-being in individuals and communities globally by embracing interdisciplinary collaboration, rigorous research approaches, and mechanistic insights into herbal actions.

CHAPTER FIVE

INVESTIGATING HERBAL CONCOCTIONS AND USES

Applications and formulations of herbs include a wide range of goods and preparations made from botanical extracts and medicinal plants. Herbal formulations are used for many medical, cosmetic, gastronomic, and cultural purposes; they range from conventional treatments to cutting-edge inventions. We will explore the various kinds of herbal preparations, topical treatments, herbal supplements and nutraceuticals, herbal personal care items and cosmetics, and the culinary and gastronomic uses of medicinal plants in this comprehensive analysis.

Herbal Concoctions, Decoctions, and Tinctures

Herbal preparations are ways to take the medicinal ingredients present in medicinal plants and use them for improving or treating health. The extraction techniques, solvents employed, and intended uses differ amongst them. The following are a few typical herbal remedies:

1. Infusions: Dried or fresh herbs are steeped in hot water to extract the active ingredients in infusions, commonly referred to as herbal teas or tisanes. Traditionally, infusions are made by covering herbs with boiling water, letting them steep for a predetermined amount of time, and then filtering. They can be drunk as a tasty beverage or taken internally for their therapeutic qualities. Examples of herbal infusions include chamomile tea, peppermint tea, and ginger tea.

2. Decoctions: While decoctions and infusions are similar, decoctions extract the therapeutic ingredients from herbs by simmering them in water over low heat. Stronger plant components like seeds, bark, and roots that need to be heated for a lengthy time to release their active ingredients are typically decoctions. The liquid is filtered and drunk after it has simmered. In conventional herbal treatment systems like Traditional Chinese treatment (TCM) and Ayurveda, decoctions are frequently utilized.

3. Tinctures: Made by macerating herbs in alcohol or a combination of alcohol and water, tinctures are

concentrated liquid extracts. In order to extract the bioactive chemicals from the plants and create a strong, shelf-stable formulation, alcohol is used as a solvent. Usually, tinctures are taken orally after being diluted in juice or water. They are prized for their capacity to maintain the therapeutic qualities of herbs as well as their lengthy shelf life and simplicity of dosage. Ginkgo biloba, valerian, and echinacea are common herbs used in tinctures.

External Uses: Oils, Salves, and Poultices

Medicinal herbs are used internally as well as externally in a variety of ways to treat musculoskeletal diseases, wounds, and skin conditions. Herbs can be applied externally as liniments, oils, salves, creams, and poultices. Here are a few instances:

1.Poultices: Poultices are herbal concoctions applied topically as a moist or dry compress. They are created by crushing or grinding dried or fresh herbs. Poultices are applied topically to reduce swelling, ease pain, encourage the healing of wounds, and extract poisons from the body. Calendula flowers, comfrey root, and plantain leaves are common poultice materials. In order to keep them in place, poultices are usually wrapped with a cloth or bandage and applied either warm or cold.

2.Oils: Dried or fresh herbs are steeped in a carrier oil, like almond, coconut, or olive oil, to create infused oils called herbal oils. To extract the therapeutic components of the herbs, they are let to macerate in the oil for a few weeks. Herbal oils can be used topically on the skin for skincare, massage, and aromatherapy. Their soothing, hydrating, and nourishing qualities make them valuable. Lavender, rosemary, and arnica oils are common herbal oils.

3.Herbal salves are semi-solid ointments that are created by combining oils infused with herbs with beeswax or other solid fats to produce a protective and calming external treatment. To treat minor burns, scratches, bug bites, and skin irritations, salves are administered topically. They provide a barrier of defense that keeps moisture in and aids in healing. Additional substances found in salves frequently include vitamin E, essential oils, and therapeutic herbs like calendula and plantain.

Supplements with Herbs and Nutraceuticals

Dietary supplements made from botanical extracts and medicinal plants are known as nutraceuticals and herbal supplements. They are employed to address particular health issues, promote general health, and prevent disease. Supplements containing herbs can be found in a variety of formats, such as liquid extracts, pills, powders, and capsules. Here are a few instances of nutraceuticals and herbal supplements:

1.Capsules and pills: For easy dosing and administration, herbal supplements are frequently crushed or encapsulated in pills. Standardized herbal extracts, powders, or a combination of herbal components may be found as capsules and tablets. They help to strengthen the immune system, facilitate better digestion, sharpen the mind, and uplift overall wellbeing.

2.Liquid Extracts: Often referred to as tinctures, liquid herbal extracts are concentrated mixtures of plant ingredients dissolved in glycerin or alcohol. Using liquid extracts to administer the medicinal qualities of plants is a practical and quick solution. They can be poured into tea, juice, or water to be consumed orally. To guarantee constant potency and effectiveness, liquid extracts are frequently standardized.

3.Herbal Powders: Dried herbs are ground into a powder and then mixed with finely ground plant ingredients to create herbal powders. For oral intake, herbal powders can be combined with juice, yogurt, water, or smoothie ingredients. They are taken as dietary supplements to boost vitality, improve sports performance, and offer nourishment. Herbal powders can also be added to bathwater for aromatherapy or used topically in skincare formulations.

Herbal Personal Care and Cosmetic Items

Herbal extracts, botanical oils, and plant-based substances are used in the production of herbal cosmetics and personal care products to nourish, cleanse, and beautify the skin, hair, and body. These products are prized for their all-natural components, mild formulas, and comprehensive skincare philosophy. Here are a few instances of herbal personal care and cosmetics products:

1. Herbal Face Cleansers: Using plant oils, herbal extracts, and natural surfactants, herbal face cleansers gently cleanse the skin while removing debris, oil, and pollutants without depleting it of its natural oils. All skin types can benefit from herbal cleansers, which are prized for their capacity to moisturize, calm, and cleanse the skin.

2. Herbal Moisturizers: Using botanical oils, humectants, and herbal extracts, herbal moisturizers replace moisture and help the skin's natural barrier function. Herbal moisturizers are used to defend against environmental harm, improve skin texture, and relieve dry, dehydrated skin. Herbal moisturizing substances including jojoba oil, aloe vera, and shea butter are commonly used.

3. Herbal Shampoos and Conditioners: Designed to wash, nourish, and fortify the hair and scalp, herbal shampoos and conditioners are hair care products formulated with herbal extracts, essential oils, and natural conditioning agents. Herbal conditioners hydrate, detangle, and soften hair while herbal shampoos gently remove oil, debris, and product

buildup without removing the natural oils from the hair. Ingredients used often in herbal hair care products include chamomile, lavender, and rosemary.

Medicinal Herbs' Applications in Cooking and Gastronomy

Medicinal herbs are utilized in culinary and gastronomic contexts to improve the flavor, aroma, and nutritional value of foods and beverages in addition to their usage in medicine and cosmetics. Essential oils, phytonutrients, and aromatic compounds give culinary herbs their distinct flavor profiles and health-promoting qualities. These components make culinary herbs valuable. Here are a few instances of how medicinal plants are used in food and cooking:

1.Herbal Infusions and Teas: Herbal infusions, teas, and herbal beverages are sometimes flavored with medicinal plants. Herbs that are valued for their aromatic oils, calming qualities, and digestive advantages include mint, chamomile, and lemon balm. Herbal teas can be made with other ingredients like honey, lemon, and spices and are consumed hot or cold.

2. Herb-Infused Oils and Vinegars: To add taste and scent to food preparations, medicinal herbs are infused into oils and vinegars. Herb-infused vinegars can be used in marinades, sauces, and dressings; herb-infused oils can be poured over salads, spaghetti, and grilled vegetables. Herb-infused oils that are commonly utilized are garlic, rosemary, and basil oils.

3. Meats and Poultry Seasoned with Herb Rubs: Spice mixes and herb rubs made from medicinal plants are used to flavor meats, poultry, and seafood. Dried herbs, spices, salt, and pepper are combined to make herb rubs, which are applied to the meat's surface before to cooking. Meats seasoned with herbs are grilled, roasted, or smoked to enhance their flavor and fragrance.

4. Desserts Flavored with Medicinal Herbs: Sweet snacks, baked goods, and desserts are flavored with medicinal herbs. Herbs like thyme, lavender, and rosemary give cakes, biscuits, and pastries a faintly flowery or herbaceous flavor. Desserts are sweetened and their flavor profiles enhanced with

the use of syrups, sugars, and extracts infused with herbs.

5.Herbal Garnishes and Decorations: To enhance the color, texture, and flavor of culinary dishes, medicinal plants are employed as garnishes and decorations. Finely chopped fresh herbs like basil, cilantro, and parsley are added as a finishing touch to soups, salads, and entrees. Cakes, beverages, and pastries are adorned with edible flowers, like violets, roses, and nasturtiums.

In summary, a broad variety of preparations and products used for culinary, cosmetic, medical, and cultural objectives are included in the formulations and applications of herbs. There are many medical, cosmetic, and culinary uses for medicinal plants, ranging from age-old cures to cutting-edge discoveries. We can take use of the healing qualities of medicinal herbs, improve our wellbeing, and savor the natural gifts that nature has to offer by investigating their many applications.

CHAPTER SIX

INVESTIGATING HERBAL MEDICINE IN PARTICULAR HEALTH CONDITIONS

Since ancient times, herbal therapy has been utilized to cure a variety of illnesses, providing all-natural solutions to go along with more traditional therapies. We will look at herbal remedies for respiratory problems, herbal remedies for digestive problems, herbal remedies for cardiovascular health, herbal remedies for immune system support, and herbal remedies for neurological ailments in this in-depth analysis.

Herbal Remedies for Respiratory Conditions

Asthma, bronchitis, chronic obstructive pulmonary disease (COPD), and respiratory infections are among the ailments that fall under the category of respiratory disorders. These conditions impact the lungs, airways, and respiratory system. Herbal therapy provides a range of methods to promote respiratory health and reduce these illnesses' related symptoms:

1.Herbal expectorants: Herbs that assist loosen and remove mucus from the respiratory tract, such as mullein (Verbascum thapsus), elecampane (Inula helenium), and thyme (Thymus vulgaris), facilitate coughing and help clear the airways. These herbs are frequently used to treat respiratory pain, coughing, and congestion.

2.Herbs known as bronchodilators, like lobelia (Lobelia inflata), peppermint (Mentha × piperita), and eucalyptus (Eucalyptus globulus), relieve respiratory symptoms like wheezing and shortness of breath by relaxing the bronchial muscles and opening up the airways.

3.Anti-inflammatory Herbs: Herbs that reduce inflammation in the respiratory tract, reduce swelling, and enhance breathing function in conditions like asthma and bronchitis include licorice (Glycyrrhiza glabra), boswellia (Boswellia serrata), and ginger (Zingiber officinale).

4.Immune-Supportive Herbs: By boosting immune function and lessening the intensity and duration of symptoms, immune-supportive herbs like echinacea (Echinacea purpurea), astragalus (Astragalus membranaceus), and elderberry (Sambucus nigra) help to strengthen the immune system and protect against respiratory infections.

5.Antimicrobial Herbs: With their ability to inhibit the growth of bacteria, viruses, and fungi in the respiratory tract, antimicrobial herbs like thyme (Thymus vulgaris), garlic (Allium sativum), and oregano (Origanum vulgare) help to support respiratory health and lower the risk of respiratory infections.

Herbal Treatment of Intestinal Illnesses

A variety of illnesses affecting the gastrointestinal tract are referred to as digestive disorders. These conditions include gastritis, indigestion, heartburn, irritable bowel syndrome (IBS), and inflammatory bowel disease (IBD). Herbal medicine provides a range of methods to promote intestinal health and reduce symptoms related to certain conditions:

1.Digestive Bitters: Herbs that are bitter, like dandelion (Taraxacum officinale), artichoke (Cynara cardunculus), and gentian (Gentiana lutea), increase the production of digestive juices, such as bile, stomach acid, and enzymes. This improves digestion, eases indigestion, and encourages gastrointestinal motility.

2.Carminative Herbs: By relaxing intestinal muscles, releasing trapped gas, and calming digestive spasms, carminative herbs including ginger (Zingiber officinale), fennel (Foeniculum vulgare), and peppermint (Mentha × piperita) assist to relieve gas, bloating, and abdominal pain.

3.Anti-inflammatory Herbs: Herbs that reduce inflammation in the gastrointestinal tract, ease discomfort, and promote healing in illnesses including gastritis, IBS, and IBD include marshmallow (Althaea officinalis), chamomile (Matricaria chamomilla), and turmeric (Curcuma longa).

4.Herbs that Calm the Gut: Herbs that calm the gut lining include marshmallow (Althaea officinalis), licorice (Glycyrrhiza glabra), and slippery elm (Ulmus rubra). These herbs create a mucilaginous layer that soothes the gastrointestinal tract's lining and guards against irritation, inflammation, and ulcers.

5.Probiotic Herbs: Plants rich in beneficial bacteria that aid in the growth of the gut flora, microbial balance restoration, and immune system and digestive health include chamomile (Matricaria chamomilla), lemon balm (Melissa officinalis), and peppermint (Mentha × piperita).

Herbal Therapy to Promote Heart Health

The state of the heart, blood vessels, and circulatory system are all included in cardiovascular health. Numerous strategies to promote cardiovascular health and lower the risk of cardiovascular disorders such excessive blood pressure, high cholesterol, and heart disease are available with herbal medicine:

1.Herbs that are cardiotonic: Herbs that are cardiotonic include motherwort (Leonurus cardiaca), garlic (Allium sativum), and hawthorn (Crataegus spp.). These herbs aid to improve cardiac function, strengthen the heart muscle, and regulate blood pressure and circulation.

2.Herbs known as vasodilators, such ginkgo (Ginkgo biloba), ginger (Zingiber officinale), and hawthorn (Crataegus spp.), serve to relax and widen the blood vessels, which improves blood flow, lowers blood pressure, and improves circulation.

3.Herbs that Lower Blood Pressure: By promoting vasodilation, reducing vascular resistance, and inhibiting the renin-angiotensin-aldosterone system, antihypertensive herbs like garlic (Allium sativum), olive leaf (Olea europaea), and celery seed (Apium graveolens) help lower blood pressure, reduce hypertension, and protect against cardiovascular disease.

4.Antioxidant Herbs: Herbs high in antioxidants, such green tea (Camellia sinensis), hawthorn (Crataegus spp.), and turmeric (Curcuma longa), aid to prevent inflammation and cardiovascular disease by reducing oxidative stress and free radical damage.

5.Anticoagulant Herbs: Anticoagulant herbs can assist to enhance blood flow, lower the risk of thrombosis, stroke, and cardiovascular events, and prevent blood clot formation. Examples of these herbs are ginkgo (Ginkgo biloba), garlic (Allium sativum), and ginger (Zingiber officinale).

Using Herbs to Boost the Immune System

Strategies to strengthen immunity, increase resistance to infections, and advance general health and wellbeing are all included in immune support. Herbal medicine provides a range of methods to bolster the body's defenses and enhance immunological function:

1.Herbs that modulate immune function: Herbs that modulate immune function include echinacea (Echinacea purpurea), astragalus (Astragalus membranaceus), and medicinal mushrooms (reishi, shiitake, and maitake). They also support immune responses to infections and pathogens.

2.Adaptogenic Herbs: Herbs that help regulate and strengthen the body's stress response systems, improve resilience to stress, and boost immunological function include rhodiola (Rhodiola rosea), holy basil (Ocimum sanctum), and ashwagandha (Withania somnifera).

3.Antiviral Herbs: Herbs that limit viral replication, strengthen immune systems, and lessen the severity and duration of viral illnesses, such as colds, the flu, and respiratory viruses, include licorice (Glycyrrhiza glabra), olive leaf (Olea europaea), and elderberry (Sambucus nigra).

4.Antibacterial Herbs: Plants that prevent the growth of dangerous bacteria, support microbial balance, and fortify immune systems against bacterial infections include garlic (Allium sativum), oregano (Origanum vulgare), and thyme (Thymus vulgaris).

5.Antioxidant Herbs: By shielding immune cells from harm and boosting their activity, antioxidant herbs like rosemary (Rosmarinus officinalis), green tea (Camellia sinensis), and turmeric (Curcuma longa) aid to neutralize free radicals, lower oxidative stress, and promote immunological function.

Herbal Remedies for Nervous System Disorders

A variety of ailments involving the brain, spinal cord, and peripheral nerves are referred to as neurological conditions. These disorders include depression, anxiety, insomnia, migraines, and neurodegenerative diseases including Parkinson's and Alzheimer's.

Herbal medicine provides a range of methods to promote neurological health and reduce symptoms related to these illnesses:

1. Anxiolytic Herbs: By modifying neurotransmitter activity and GABAergic signaling, anxiolytic herbs like valerian (Valeriana officinalis), kava (Piper methysticum), and passionflower (Passiflora incarnata) aid to reduce anxiety, calm the nervous system, and induce relaxation.

2. Antidepressant Herbs: By raising serotonin and dopamine levels and modifying neurotransmitter function, antidepressant herbs like rhodiola (Rhodiola rosea), saffron (Crocus sativus), and St. John's wort (Hypericum perforatum) help to elevate mood, improve emotional well-being, and lessen symptoms of depression.

3. Herbs that promote relaxation, enhance sleep-wake regulation, and lessen insomnia include chamomile (Matricaria chamomilla), lemon balm (Melissa officinalis), and hops (Humulus lupulus). These herbs also promote GABAergic neurotransmission.

4.Analgesic Herbs: By inhibiting prostaglandin synthesis, modulating pain receptors, and blocking pain signals, analgesic herbs like feverfew (Tanacetum parthenium), willow bark (Salix spp.), and Jamaican dogwood (Piscidia piscipula) help to relieve pain, reduce inflammation, and alleviate migraine symptoms.

5.Neuroprotective Herbs: By lowering oxidative stress, preventing neuroinflammation, and encouraging neuronal repair and regeneration, neuroprotective herbs like ginkgo (Ginkgo biloba), turmeric (Curcuma longa), and bacopa (Bacopa monnieri) help to protect against neurodegenerative diseases, support cognitive function, and enhance brain health.

To sum up, herbal medicine provides a multitude of therapeutic alternatives for treating a variety of medical diseases, including digestive, respiratory, immunological, and neurological illnesses. People can improve their overall health and well-being, support their body's natural healing processes, and encourage long-term health and vitality by integrating herbal treatments into comprehensive treatment plans. To guarantee safety and effectiveness, it is imperative that you speak with a licensed healthcare professional prior to utilizing herbal treatments, particularly if you are on medication or have pre-existing medical issues.

CHAPTER SEVEN

GETTING AROUND THE LAW AND REGULATION FOR HERBAL PRODUCTS

Due to their ability to provide natural solutions for a wide range of health issues, herbal products hold a prominent position in healthcare systems across the globe. Nonetheless, the laws and regulations pertaining to herbal products are intricate and varied. We will examine the global regulation of herbal products, sound manufacturing practices and quality control, traditional knowledge and intellectual property rights, marketing ethics for herbal products, and consumer safety in herbal medicine in this in-depth investigation.

Global Herbal Product Regulation

Countries have very different regulations on herbal products because of things like historical usage, cultural customs, safety concerns, and changing scientific knowledge. While some nations have strict laws governing herbal items, others have less stringent laws or disjointed regulations. Below is a summary of the regulatory frameworks that are widely used across the globe:

1.Traditional Medical Systems: Ayurveda, Unani, and Traditional Chinese Medicine (TCM) are just a few of the wealthy nations that have developed regulatory structures to control the manufacturing, exportation, and application of herbal remedies. Regulatory guidelines are frequently infused with conventional knowledge, diagnostic techniques, and therapeutic ideas by means of these frameworks.

2.Pharmaceutical Regulations: Herbal products are subject to strict safety, effectiveness, quality control, and labeling regulations in some countries where they are controlled as pharmaceuticals. Herbal medicine manufacturers must follow Good Manufacturing Practices (GMP) and carry out clinical research to confirm the products' safety and efficacy before they are authorized for sale and marketing.

3.Dietary Supplements: Compared to pharmaceuticals, herbal products are subject to less restrictive restrictions in many countries where they are classified as food products or dietary supplements. The main goals of dietary supplement laws are usually to guarantee product quality, safety, and correct labeling. But before dietary supplements are sold, their effectiveness might not be well assessed.

4.Traditional Herbal Medicines: In recognition of the historical and cultural value of traditional herbal medicines, many nations have set up distinct regulatory paths for them. These regulatory frameworks, which demand manufacturers to present proof of safety, efficacy, and quality based on conventional use and/or scientific research, frequently strike a compromise between conventional wisdom and contemporary scientific data.

5.Herbal Cosmetics: In some states, topical herbal products—like creams, lotions, and shampoos—may be subject to regulations similar to those governing cosmetics. Cosmetic rules do not prioritize therapeutic or efficacious claims; instead, they center on product safety, labeling, and advertising claims.

6.Online Sales of Herbal items: Since online sales of herbal items may elude traditional regulatory scrutiny, the growth of e-commerce has presented new regulatory concerns. Certain nations have put in place policies to keep an eye on and control the online sales of herbal goods. These policies include demands for standards for product labeling, advertising, and registration.

QA and GMPs (good manufacturing practices)

The safety, effectiveness, and quality of herbal products are contingent upon the implementation of quality assurance and good manufacturing principles (GMP). GMP regulations give producers a framework for upholding constant quality requirements from the procurement of raw materials to the distribution of the finished product. Important elements of GMP for herbal products include of:

1.Purchasing Raw Materials: In order to guarantee the authenticity, purity, and quality of their raw materials, manufacturers must pick and procure them from reliable vendors with care. This could entail carrying out identity checks, determining whether pollutants are present, and confirming compliance with sustainable and ethical sourcing guidelines.

2.Production Procedures: In order to guarantee the consistency, cleanliness, and safety of the product, GMP laws specify particular standards for production facilities, tools, and procedures. This entails putting quality control measures into place, creating standardized operating procedures (SOPs), and keeping accurate records of production activities.

3.Quality Control Testing: Throughout the production process, herbal products are subjected to stringent quality control testing to confirm their identity, safety, potency, and purity. This could entail conducting analytical testing to find impurities, guarantee consistency, and verify adherence to standards using techniques including chromatography, spectroscopy, and microbiological assays.

4.Product Labeling and Packaging: In accordance with GMP guidelines, herbal goods must bear accurate labels that give consumers access to critical details such component lists, dosage guidelines, expiration dates, and storage advice. In order to prevent contamination, deterioration, and tampering with herbal goods during storage and transit, proper packaging is also essential.

5.Post-Market Surveillance: After herbal goods are introduced to the market, manufacturers are required to put in place mechanisms for post-market surveillance to keep an eye on their quality and safety. This could entail product recalls, adverse event reporting, and continuous quality testing to find and fix any potential problems.

Traditional Knowledge and Intellectual Property Rights

In the herbal products sector, protecting intellectual property rights (IPR) and traditional knowledge (TK) is a complicated and divisive topic, especially when it comes to the marketing of traditional herbal treatments and native plant resources. Important things to think about are:

1.Patents and Trademarks: In order to safeguard their intellectual property and obtain the sole right to market and sell these items, businesses may apply for patents or trademarks for innovative herbal formulations, extraction techniques, or product compositions. However, there has been discussion and controversy around the patenting of indigenous plant resources or traditional herbal medicines. This is especially true when the patents are thought to be biopiracy or misuse of traditional knowledge.

2.Protection of Traditional Knowledge: Oral traditions and cultural practices have allowed indigenous groups and traditional healers to pass down invaluable knowledge about the therapeutic qualities of plants over the decades. In order to preserve traditional knowledge, measures for benefit-sharing and fair access to genetic resources must be put in place, as well as recognition of indigenous rights and communal ownership of TK.

3.Access and Benefit-Sharing (ABS): The goal of the Nagoya Protocol, an addendum to the Convention on Biological Diversity (CBD), is to encourage just and equitable distribution of the advantages that come from using traditional knowledge and genetic resources. The purpose of ABS agreements is to make sure that the communities who have helped to develop and conserve herbal products share in the benefits that come with their commercialization.

4.Ethical Engagement: Businesses that market herbal products have an obligation to interact ethically with indigenous people, honor their cultural legacy and traditional knowledge, and obtain their cooperation and informed consent before gaining access to genetic resources or conventional medical knowledge. Respecting indigenous rights, encouraging cultural awareness, and developing mutually beneficial relationships built on reciprocity and trust are examples of ethical principles.

Marketing Herbal Products with Integrity

Promoting to customers accurate, truthful, and transparent information regarding the efficacy, safety, and quality of herbal goods is a key component of ethical marketing. Important moral factors in the promotion of herbal products are as follows:

1.Honest Labeling and Advertising: Businesses need to make sure that information regarding the ingredients, advantages, and possible drawbacks of herbal products is accurately provided on product labels, packaging, and advertising materials. It is best to stay away from making false or misleading marketing claims, such as those that make unsubstantiated therapeutic claims or exaggerated health advantages.

2.Consent Based on Information: Patients are entitled to information regarding the healthcare options available to them, including the use of herbal remedies. To help consumers make educated decisions, businesses should make information on possible side effects, contraindications, and interactions with other medications or medical conditions explicit and easily accessible.

3.Scientific Validation: Claims made in marketing for herbal products should be backed up by facts from traditional uses, clinical trials, and pharmacological research, if relevant. Businesses should refrain from promoting their products with unsupported claims or anecdotal proof only.

4.Responsible Endorsement: Businesses should use caution when asking influencers, celebrities, or medical professionals to promote herbal products. They should also make sure that the endorsements are grounded in factual knowledge, empirical data, and moral considerations. Endorsements must not deceive customers or suggest unjustified health benefits.

5.Social Responsibility: Beyond just following the law, ethical marketing strategies take into account a wider range of social responsibility issues. Examples of these include fair trade policies, environmentally friendly products, and CSR programs that strengthen ethical supply chains and benefit local communities.

Herbal medicine and consumer safety

Given the possible risks of incorrect usage, contamination, adulteration, and combinations with other pharmaceuticals, consumer safety is of utmost importance when it comes to the regulation and use of herbal medicine. The following are important factors to ensure customer safety:

1.Quality Control: To guarantee the security, effectiveness, and purity of herbal products, manufacturers are required to follow strict quality control procedures. This entails confirming the legitimacy and identity of raw materials in addition to testing for pollutants, heavy metals, pesticides, and microbial contamination.

2.Adverse Event Reporting: Systems for reporting adverse events, such as allergic responses, side effects, and interactions, connected to herbal products should be available to both consumers and medical experts. Regulatory bodies utilize this data to keep an eye on the safety of products and to take the necessary precautions to safeguard the public's health.

3.Drug-Herb Interactions: Herbal supplements, over-the-counter medicines, and prescription drugs may interact with herbal products to cause negative side effects or diminished efficacy. Before utilizing herbal products, consumers should speak with healthcare providers, particularly if they are on medication or have underlying medical issues.

4.Product Labeling: The dosage, directions for administration, possible side effects, contraindications, and precautions should all be clearly and accurately stated on the labels of herbal products. This lowers the possibility of abuse or unfavorable reactions and gives customers the power to choose products wisely.

5.Education and knowledge: To ensure the safe and responsible use of herbal products, it is imperative to promote consumer education and knowledge about herbal medicine, including its benefits, hazards, and proper use. This involves giving patients and healthcare providers access to trustworthy data, tools, and educational materials.

In summary, managing the legal and regulatory environment surrounding herbal products necessitates a thorough comprehension of international laws, quality control procedures, intellectual property rights, moral marketing concepts, and consumer safety issues. Promoting openness, responsibility, and moral behavior across the herbal goods sector will allow stakeholders to protect the integrity of herbal medicine and guarantee that people all over the world have safe and efficient access to natural healthcare solutions.

www.ingramcontent.com/pod-product-compliance
Lightning Source LLC
Chambersburg PA
CBHW070156230526
45471CB00002B/691